THE ANEMIA DIET BIBLE

Healthy Foods To Fight Anemia And Nourishing Recipes To Increase Your Iron And Energy Levels For Beginners

CRUE GAGE

Copyright © 2024 By Crue Gage

All Rights Reserved.

Table of Contents

Introductory 5

CHAPTER ONE 14

   Impact On Health And Well-Being 14

   Nutritional Needs For Anemia & Foods To Include 20

CHAPTER TWO 24

   Sample Foods And Meals 24

   Foods To Avoid Or Limit 27

   Principles Of Anemia-Friendly Meal Planning 31

   Sample Meal Plan 35

CHAPTER THREE 37

   Breakfast Recipes 37

   Lunch Recipes 43

   Dinner Recipes 51

   Snack And Smoothie Recipes 59

CHAPTER FOUR 69

   Cooking Tips To Maximize Nutrient Retention 69

   Combining Foods For Optimal Nutrient Absorption 75

CHAPTER FIVE 83

Managing Anemia With Vegetarian And Vegan Diets 83

Hydration And Its Role In Anemia Management 92

CHAPTER SIX' 99

When To Consider Supplements & Choosing The Right Supplements 99

Tracking Symptoms And Progress 108

Regular Blood Tests And What They Mean 116

CHAPTER SEVEN 126

Adjusting Your Diet Based On Test Results 126

THE END 136

Introductory

Anemia is a medical condition that is defined by a deficiency in the quantity or quality of red blood cells (RBCs) or in the quantity of hemoglobin, the protein inside RBCs that transports oxygen throughout the body. This deficiency can result in a variety of health issues and symptoms by reducing the delivery of oxygen to the body's tissues and organs.

Types of Anemia:

- **Iron-Deficiency Anemia**: The most common type, caused by a lack of iron, which is necessary for hemoglobin production.

- **Vitamin-Deficiency Anemia**: Caused by a deficiency in vitamins needed for RBC production, such as vitamin B12 or folate.

- **Aplastic Anemia**: A rare condition where the bone marrow fails to produce enough RBCs.

- **Hemolytic Anemia**: Occurs when RBCs are destroyed faster than they can be produced.

- **Sickle Cell Anemia**: A genetic disorder where RBCs are misshapen, leading to various complications.

- **Thalassemia**: A genetic disorder affecting hemoglobin production.

- **Chronic Disease Anemia**: Associated with chronic diseases that affect RBC production, such as cancer or HIV/AIDS.

Symptoms of Anemia:

- Fatigue
- Weakness
- Pale or yellowish skin
- Shortness of breath
- Dizziness or lightheadedness
- Cold hands and feet
- Chest pain
- Headaches

Causes of Anemia:

- Blood loss (e.g., heavy menstrual periods, gastrointestinal bleeding)
- Nutritional deficiencies (e.g., iron, vitamin B12, folate)
- Chronic diseases (e.g., kidney disease, rheumatoid arthritis)
- Genetic disorders (e.g., sickle cell anemia, thalassemia)

- Bone marrow disorders
- Infections

Diagnosis and Treatment:

- **Diagnosis**: Anemia is typically diagnosed through blood tests, including a complete blood count (CBC) to measure hemoglobin levels and the number of RBCs. Other tests may be conducted to determine the underlying cause.

  - **Treatment**: The treatment of anemia depends on its cause:
  - **Iron supplements** for iron-deficiency anemia.
  - **Vitamin B12 or folate supplements** for vitamin-deficiency anemia.
  - **Medications** to stimulate RBC production or treat underlying conditions.

- **Blood transfusions** in severe cases.
- **Lifestyle and dietary changes** to address nutritional deficiencies.

Diet plays a crucial role in managing and preventing anemia, especially for types related to nutritional deficiencies such as iron-deficiency anemia and vitamin-deficiency anemia.

Here's how diet can help:

Iron-Rich Foods

Iron is a key component of hemoglobin, and its deficiency is a common cause of anemia. There are two types of dietary iron:

• **Heme Iron**: Found in animal products and is more easily absorbed by the body.

1. Red meat (beef, lamb)
2. Poultry (chicken, turkey)
3. Fish and seafood (salmon, tuna, shrimp)

- **Non-Heme Iron**: Found in plant-based foods and fortified products.

1. Legumes (lentils, beans, chickpeas)
2. Tofu and tempeh
3. Dark leafy greens (spinach, kale)
4. Nuts and seeds (pumpkin seeds, sesame seeds)
5. Fortified cereals and grains

Vitamin C:

- Vitamin C enhances the absorption of non-heme iron from plant-based foods. Including vitamin C-rich foods in meals can improve iron absorption.

- Citrus fruits (oranges, grapefruits)
- Berries (strawberries, raspberries)
- Tomatoes
- Bell peppers
- Broccoli and Brussels sprouts

Vitamin B12 and Folate:

• Vitamin B12 and folate are essential for RBC production. Deficiencies in these vitamins can lead to megaloblastic anemia.

Vitamin B12:

- Animal products (meat, fish, poultry, dairy)
- Fortified cereals and plant-based milks

Folate:

- Leafy green vegetables (spinach, kale)
- Legumes (lentils, beans)
- Avocado
- Fortified grains and cereals

Other Nutrients

- **Copper**: Helps with iron metabolism.
- Shellfish, seeds, nuts, organ meats
- **Vitamin A**: Plays a role in iron metabolism and hemoglobin synthesis.
- Carrots, sweet potatoes, dark leafy greens

For personalized dietary advice, especially for those with specific health conditions or dietary restrictions.

A well-balanced diet that includes these nutrients can significantly help in managing anemia and improving overall health.

CHAPTER ONE
Impact On Health And Well-Being

Anemia can have a significant impact on health and well-being, affecting various aspects of physical and mental health. Here's how anemia can influence different areas of health:

Physical Health:

- **Fatigue and Weakness**: Reduced oxygen delivery to tissues causes persistent tiredness and weakness, impacting daily activities and overall energy levels.
- **Shortness of Breath**: Inadequate oxygen levels can make breathing difficult, especially during physical exertion.
- **Pale or Yellowish Skin**: A lack of red blood cells can cause

noticeable changes in skin color, indicating reduced blood flow and oxygenation.

- **Heart Problems**: Chronic anemia can lead to an increased heart rate, heart murmurs, or even heart failure as the heart works harder to pump oxygen-rich blood.
- **Cold Hands and Feet**: Poor circulation and reduced oxygen delivery can cause a feeling of coldness in extremities.
- **Dizziness and Lightheadedness**: Low hemoglobin levels can lead to reduced blood flow to the brain, causing dizziness or fainting.
- **Immune System**: Anemia can weaken the immune system, making individuals more

susceptible to infections and illnesses.

- **Pregnancy Complications**: Pregnant women with anemia are at higher risk of complications such as preterm delivery, low birth weight, and postpartum depression.

Mental and Cognitive Health:

- **Cognitive Function**: Reduced oxygen supply to the brain can impair concentration, memory, and cognitive function, affecting academic and work performance.
- **Mood and Mental Health**: Anemia can contribute to feelings of depression, anxiety, and irritability due to chronic fatigue and poor overall health.

- **Sleep Disorders**: Symptoms like restless legs syndrome and insomnia can be exacerbated by anemia, further affecting quality of life.

Quality of Life:

- **Reduced Physical Activity**: Chronic fatigue and weakness can limit participation in physical activities, affecting fitness and overall health.
- **Social Interaction**: Persistent symptoms can lead to social withdrawal and isolation, impacting relationships and emotional well-being.
- **Work and Productivity**: Anemia can reduce productivity and

increase absenteeism due to fatigue and other health issues.

Long-Term Health:

- **Chronic Conditions**: Untreated anemia can contribute to or worsen chronic conditions such as cardiovascular disease, diabetes, and other health problems.
- **Growth and Development**: In children, anemia can impair growth and development, affecting physical and cognitive milestones.

Management and Prevention:

- **Regular Monitoring**: Regular health check-ups and blood tests can help detect and manage anemia early, preventing complications.

- **Proper Nutrition**: A balanced diet rich in essential nutrients like iron, vitamin B12, and folate can help prevent anemia and improve overall health.
- **Medical Treatment**: Adhering to prescribed treatments and medications can effectively manage anemia and reduce its impact on health.
- **Lifestyle Adjustments**: Incorporating healthy lifestyle habits such as regular exercise, adequate sleep, and stress management can improve well-being and mitigate anemia symptoms.

By addressing anemia through appropriate medical treatment and lifestyle changes, individuals can significantly improve their health, well-being, and quality of life.

Nutritional Needs For Anemia & Foods To Include

For managing anemia, meeting specific nutritional needs is essential to boost red blood cell production and improve overall health. Here's a guide to the key nutrients needed and the foods that can help:

Key Nutrients and Their Sources:

Iron:

- **Heme Iron** (more easily absorbed):

    1. Red meat (beef, lamb)
    2. Poultry (chicken, turkey)
    3. Fish and seafood (salmon, tuna, shrimp)

- **Non-Heme Iron** (plant-based):

1. Lentils and beans (black beans, chickpeas)
2. Tofu and tempeh
3. Dark leafy greens (spinach, kale)
4. Nuts and seeds (pumpkin seeds, sunflower seeds)
5. Fortified cereals and grains (oatmeal, whole-grain bread)

Vitamin C:

1. Enhances non-heme iron absorption:
2. Citrus fruits (oranges, grapefruits)
3. Berries (strawberries, raspberries)
4. Bell peppers
5. Tomatoes
6. Broccoli and Brussels sprouts

Vitamin B12:

1. Essential for red blood cell production:
2. Animal products (meat, fish, poultry, dairy products)
3. Fortified plant-based milks and cereals
4. Eggs

Folate (Vitamin B9):

1. Crucial for DNA synthesis and RBC production:
2. Leafy green vegetables (spinach, kale)
3. Legumes (lentils, beans)
4. Avocado
5. Fortified grains and cereals
6. Beets

Copper:

1. Aids in iron metabolism:

2. Shellfish (oysters, crab)
3. Nuts and seeds (sunflower seeds, cashews)
4. Whole grains (quinoa, barley)
5. Dark chocolate

Vitamin A:

1. Supports iron metabolism and overall health:
2. Carrots
3. Sweet potatoes
4. Dark leafy greens (kale, spinach)
5. Red and yellow bell peppers

CHAPTER TWO
Sample Foods And Meals

Breakfast:

- Fortified cereal with milk (iron and B12) and a side of orange slices (vitamin C)
- Smoothie with spinach, berries, and a scoop of fortified protein powder

Lunch:

- Salad with dark leafy greens, chickpeas, bell peppers, and a lemon-tahini dressing
- Turkey or chicken sandwich on whole-grain bread with a side of fruit

Dinner:

- Grilled salmon with quinoa and steamed broccoli
- Beef stir-fry with mixed vegetables (including bell peppers) over brown rice

Snacks:

- Apple slices with almond butter
- Greek yogurt with a handful of nuts and seeds

Tips for Maximizing Nutrient Absorption:

- **Combine Iron with Vitamin C**: Eating foods rich in vitamin C alongside iron-rich foods enhances absorption.
- **Avoid Inhibitors**: Minimize consumption of tea, coffee, and high-calcium foods during iron-

rich meals, as they can inhibit iron absorption.

- **Prepare Foods Thoughtfully**: For plant-based sources of iron, methods like soaking, fermenting, or sprouting can help increase iron absorption.

By including a variety of these nutrient-rich foods in your diet, you can effectively support red blood cell production, improve iron levels, and manage anemia more effectively.

Foods To Avoid Or Limit

When managing anemia, it's important to be mindful of foods and substances that can inhibit iron absorption or otherwise affect overall nutrient balance. Here are some foods and factors to avoid or limit:

Foods and Substances That Inhibit Iron Absorption:

Coffee and Tea:

• Contain compounds called polyphenols and tannins that can inhibit the absorption of both heme and non-heme iron. It's best to consume these beverages between meals rather than with meals.

Calcium-Rich Foods:

• High calcium intake, particularly from supplements or large amounts of dairy products, can interfere with iron absorption. If you need calcium supplements, take them at a different time from iron-rich meals.

High-Fiber Foods:

• Foods high in fiber, such as bran and whole grains, contain phytates that can bind iron and reduce its absorption. While fiber is an important part of a healthy diet, consuming it in moderation and balancing it with iron-rich foods can help.

Phytate-Rich Foods:

• Phytates, found in whole grains, legumes, nuts, and seeds, can inhibit iron absorption. Soaking, fermenting, or sprouting these foods can reduce their phytate content.

Oxalate-Rich Foods:

- Foods high in oxalates, such as spinach, rhubarb, and beet greens, can also inhibit iron absorption. While these foods are nutritious, they should be balanced with other iron-rich foods.

Foods to Limit:

Processed Foods:

- Highly processed foods often lack essential nutrients and may not provide the necessary vitamins and minerals needed for managing anemia.

High-Sugar Foods:

- Foods high in added sugars can contribute to poor overall nutritional status and may not provide the essential nutrients needed for optimal health.

Foods High in Sodium:

- Excessive sodium can lead to health problems such as high blood pressure, which can indirectly affect overall well-being. Limiting high-sodium foods can contribute to better overall health.

Tips for Managing Food Intake

- **Balance Your Diet**: Ensure that your diet is well-balanced with a variety of nutrient-rich foods, including those that enhance iron absorption.
- **Timing of Meals**: If consuming iron-rich foods, try to eat them at times when you're not consuming inhibitors like coffee, tea, or high-calcium foods.
- **Consult with a Healthcare Professional**: For personalized advice and guidance, particularly if

you have specific dietary restrictions or health conditions.

By being aware of these factors and making mindful dietary choices, you can optimize iron absorption and effectively manage anemia.

Principles Of Anemia-Friendly Meal Planning

Meal planning for anemia involves creating balanced, nutrient-rich meals that support red blood cell production and enhance iron absorption. Here are some principles to follow:

1. Include Iron-Rich Foods:

- **Heme Iron Sources**: Incorporate lean meats, poultry, and fish into your meals. These sources provide the most readily absorbed form of iron.

- **Non-Heme Iron Sources**: Add plant-based sources like legumes, tofu, dark leafy greens, and fortified cereals. Combine these with vitamin C-rich foods to boost absorption.

2. Enhance Iron Absorption:

- **Pair with Vitamin C**: Include foods high in vitamin C (e.g., citrus fruits, bell peppers, broccoli) in meals with iron-rich foods to improve non-heme iron absorption.
- **Avoid Inhibitors**: Minimize consumption of coffee, tea, and high-calcium foods around

mealtimes to prevent interference with iron absorption.

3. Balance with Essential Nutrients:

- **Vitamin B12 and Folate**: Ensure your diet includes foods rich in vitamin B12 (e.g., meat, dairy, fortified cereals) and folate (e.g., leafy greens, legumes), which are crucial for red blood cell production.
- **Copper and Vitamin A**: Incorporate copper-rich foods (e.g., shellfish, nuts) and vitamin A-rich foods (e.g., carrots, sweet potatoes) to support overall blood health.

4. Plan Balanced Meals:

- **Variety**: Aim for a variety of nutrient-dense foods in each meal to cover all essential vitamins and minerals.
- **Portion Control**: Manage portion sizes to include appropriate amounts of each nutrient-rich food without overloading on any single type.

5. Incorporate Nutrient-Dense Snacks:

- **Healthy Snacks**: Choose snacks that provide additional iron and other essential nutrients, such as a handful of nuts and seeds, fortified cereal with milk, or a fruit smoothie with spinach.

Work with a healthcare provider or dietitian to tailor your meal plan to your specific health needs and dietary restrictions.

Sample Meal Plan

Breakfast:

• Oatmeal fortified with iron, topped with fresh strawberries and a side of scrambled eggs (provides iron, vitamin C, and B12).

Lunch:

• Spinach and chickpea salad with bell peppers, cherry tomatoes, and a lemon-tahini dressing (iron, vitamin C, folate).

Snack:

• Greek yogurt with a sprinkle of pumpkin seeds and a small orange (calcium, iron, vitamin C).

Dinner:

• Grilled salmon with quinoa and steamed broccoli (heme iron, folate, vitamin C).

Dessert:

• Fresh fruit salad with kiwi and kiwi-based smoothie (vitamin C).

By adhering to these principles, you can create an anemia-friendly meal plan that supports optimal iron levels and overall health.

CHAPTER THREE
Breakfast Recipes

Here are some anemia-friendly breakfast recipes that incorporate iron-rich ingredients and enhance absorption with vitamin C sources:

1. Spinach and Mushroom Omelette:

Ingredients:

- 2 large eggs
- 1 cup fresh spinach, chopped
- 1/2 cup mushrooms, sliced
- 1/4 cup shredded cheese (optional)
- 1 tablespoon olive oil
- Salt and pepper to taste
- 1/2 bell pepper, diced (for vitamin C)

Instructions:

- Heat olive oil in a non-stick skillet over medium heat.
- Sauté mushrooms until they are golden brown.
- Add spinach and cook until wilted.
- Whisk eggs in a bowl and pour over the spinach and mushrooms.
- Cook until eggs are set, folding the omelette in half.
- Sprinkle with cheese if desired and season with salt and pepper.
- Serve with diced bell pepper on the side for a boost of vitamin C.

2. Iron-Rich Smoothie:

Ingredients:

- 1 cup fortified plant-based milk or regular milk

- 1/2 cup Greek yogurt
- 1/2 cup frozen berries (strawberries, blueberries)
- 1 small banana
- 1 tablespoon spinach
- 1 tablespoon chia seeds
- 1 teaspoon honey (optional)

Instructions:

- Combine all ingredients in a blender.
- Blend until smooth and creamy.
- Serve immediately for a refreshing, iron-boosting breakfast.

3. Quinoa Breakfast Bowl:

Ingredients:

- 1 cup cooked quinoa
- 1/2 cup fresh strawberries, sliced

- 1/2 cup chopped kiwi (rich in vitamin C)
- 1 tablespoon flaxseeds
- 1/4 cup nuts (almonds, walnuts)
- 1 tablespoon honey or maple syrup (optional)

Instructions:

- Place cooked quinoa in a bowl.
- Top with strawberries, kiwi, and nuts.
- Drizzle with honey or maple syrup if desired.
- Sprinkle with flaxseeds and serve.

4. Fortified Cereal with Fruit

Ingredients:

- 1 cup fortified cereal (iron-fortified)
- 1 cup milk or plant-based milk

- 1/2 cup diced oranges (for vitamin C)
- 1/4 cup raisins or dried apricots (rich in iron)
- 1 tablespoon chia seeds

Instructions:

- Pour milk over cereal in a bowl.
- Top with diced oranges, raisins, and chia seeds.
- Mix gently and enjoy.

5. Avocado Toast with Bell Peppers:

Ingredients:

- 1 slice whole-grain bread
- 1/2 avocado
- 1/4 cup cherry tomatoes, halved
- 1/4 cup diced bell peppers
- Salt and pepper to taste

- 1 tablespoon lemon juice (for added vitamin C)

Instructions:

- Toast the whole-grain bread.
- Mash avocado and spread it evenly on the toast.
- Top with cherry tomatoes, bell peppers, and a sprinkle of salt and pepper.
- Drizzle with lemon juice for extra vitamin C.

These recipes incorporate iron-rich foods and pair them with vitamin C sources to enhance iron absorption, making them great choices for supporting your anemia management.

Lunch Recipes

Here are some anemia-friendly lunch recipes that combine iron-rich ingredients with vitamin C sources to help boost iron absorption:

1. Chickpea and Spinach Salad:

Ingredients:

- 1 can chickpeas, drained and rinsed
- 2 cups fresh spinach, chopped
- 1/2 cup cherry tomatoes, halved
- 1/4 cup diced red bell pepper
- 1/4 cup red onion, thinly sliced
- 1/4 cup feta cheese (optional)
- 2 tablespoons olive oil
- 1 tablespoon lemon juice
- Salt and pepper to taste

Instructions:

- In a large bowl, combine chickpeas, spinach, cherry tomatoes, bell pepper, and red onion.
- Drizzle with olive oil and lemon juice.
- Toss to combine and season with salt and pepper.
- Top with feta cheese if desired. Serve immediately or chill before serving.

2. Turkey and Veggie Wrap:

Ingredients:

- 1 whole-grain tortilla
- 3 slices turkey breast (preferably low-sodium)
- 1/2 avocado, sliced

- 1/2 cup shredded carrots
- 1/2 cup spinach or mixed greens
- 1/4 cup diced bell peppers (red or yellow for vitamin C)
- 1 tablespoon hummus or Greek yogurt (optional for spread)

Instructions:

- Spread hummus or Greek yogurt on the tortilla.
- Layer turkey slices, avocado, carrots, spinach, and bell peppers.
- Roll up the tortilla tightly and slice in half.
- Serve with a side of fruit for an extra vitamin C boost.

3. Lentil Soup:

Ingredients:

- 1 cup dried lentils, rinsed

- 1 onion, chopped
- 2 carrots, diced
- 2 celery stalks, diced
- 2 garlic cloves, minced
- 1 can diced tomatoes
- 4 cups vegetable or chicken broth
- 1 teaspoon cumin
- 1/2 teaspoon paprika
- Salt and pepper to taste
- 1 cup chopped kale or spinach (added in last 10 minutes of cooking)

Instructions:

- In a large pot, sauté onion, carrots, celery, and garlic until softened.
- Add lentils, diced tomatoes, broth, cumin, paprika, salt, and pepper.

- Bring to a boil, then reduce heat and simmer for 25-30 minutes, until lentils are tender.
- Stir in kale or spinach and cook for an additional 5 minutes.
- Serve hot, and consider adding a side of citrus fruit for a vitamin C boost.

4. Quinoa and Black Bean Salad:

Ingredients:

- 1 cup cooked quinoa
- 1 can black beans, drained and rinsed
- 1/2 cup corn kernels (fresh or frozen)
- 1/2 cup diced cherry tomatoes
- 1/4 cup diced red onion
- 1/4 cup chopped cilantro
- 2 tablespoons olive oil

- 1 tablespoon lime juice (for vitamin C)
- Salt and pepper to taste

Instructions:

- In a large bowl, combine quinoa, black beans, corn, cherry tomatoes, red onion, and cilantro.
- Drizzle with olive oil and lime juice.
- Toss gently to combine and season with salt and pepper.
- Serve chilled or at room temperature.

5. Stuffed Bell Peppers:

Ingredients:

- 4 bell peppers (any color)
- 1 cup cooked brown rice or quinoa

- 1/2 cup cooked ground turkey or beef (optional)
- 1/2 cup black beans
- 1/2 cup corn kernels
- 1/2 cup diced tomatoes
- 1/2 cup shredded cheese (optional)
- 1 teaspoon cumin
- Salt and pepper to taste

Instructions:

- Preheat oven to 375°F (190°C).
- Cut the tops off the bell peppers and remove seeds.
- In a bowl, mix cooked rice or quinoa, ground meat (if using), black beans, corn, tomatoes, cheese (if using), cumin, salt, and pepper.

- Stuff the bell peppers with the mixture and place in a baking dish.
- Cover with foil and bake for 30 minutes. Remove foil and bake for an additional 10 minutes until peppers are tender.
- Serve warm.

These lunch recipes incorporate iron-rich ingredients and vitamin C sources to support effective anemia management while providing delicious and nutritious options for your daily meals.

Dinner Recipes

Here are some anemia-friendly dinner recipes that feature iron-rich ingredients and vitamin C sources to help boost iron absorption:

1. Grilled Salmon with Quinoa and Steamed Broccoli:

Ingredients:

- 2 salmon fillets
- 1 tablespoon olive oil
- 1 lemon, sliced
- 1 teaspoon dried dill or fresh dill
- Salt and pepper to taste
- 1 cup quinoa, rinsed
- 2 cups water or vegetable broth
- 2 cups broccoli florets

Instructions:

- Preheat the grill or oven to 400°F (200°C).
- Brush salmon fillets with olive oil, season with dill, salt, and pepper. Place lemon slices on top.
- Grill or bake for 10-15 minutes, or until salmon is cooked through.
- Cook quinoa according to package instructions, using water or broth for extra flavor.
- Steam broccoli until tender (about 5-7 minutes).
- Serve salmon over quinoa with steamed broccoli on the side.

2. Chicken and Sweet Potato Skillet:

Ingredients:

- 2 chicken breasts, diced
- 2 tablespoons olive oil

- 1 large sweet potato, peeled and diced
- 1 red bell pepper, diced (for vitamin C)
- 1 cup baby spinach or kale
- 1 teaspoon paprika
- 1/2 teaspoon garlic powder
- Salt and pepper to taste

Instructions:

- Heat olive oil in a large skillet over medium heat.
- Add chicken and cook until browned and cooked through, about 6-8 minutes.
- Add diced sweet potato, paprika, garlic powder, salt, and pepper. Cook, stirring occasionally, until sweet potatoes are tender, about 10-12 minutes.

- Stir in red bell pepper and cook for another 2-3 minutes.
- Add spinach or kale and cook until wilted.
- Serve hot.

3. Beef and Vegetable Stir-Fry:

Ingredients:

- 1 lb beef sirloin, thinly sliced
- 2 tablespoons soy sauce
- 1 tablespoon hoisin sauce
- 1 tablespoon olive oil or sesame oil
- 1 cup snap peas
- 1 cup bell peppers (any color), sliced
- 1/2 cup broccoli florets
- 1 garlic clove, minced
- 1 tablespoon grated ginger

- Cooked brown rice or quinoa for serving

Instructions:

- In a bowl, marinate beef with soy sauce and hoisin sauce for 15 minutes.
- Heat oil in a large skillet or wok over high heat.
- Add beef and cook until browned, about 3-4 minutes. Remove and set aside.
- In the same skillet, add garlic and ginger, and cook for 30 seconds.
- Add snap peas, bell peppers, and broccoli. Stir-fry for 4-5 minutes until vegetables are tender-crisp.
- Return beef to the skillet and stir to combine. Cook for another 2 minutes.

- Serve over brown rice or quinoa.

4. Stuffed Portobello Mushrooms:

Ingredients:

- 4 large portobello mushrooms
- 1 cup cooked farro or quinoa
- 1/2 cup diced tomatoes
- 1/4 cup chopped black olives
- 1/4 cup chopped onions
- 1/4 cup crumbled feta cheese (optional)
- 2 tablespoons olive oil
- 1 teaspoon dried oregano
- Salt and pepper to taste

Instructions:

- Preheat oven to 375°F (190°C).
- Remove stems and gills from portobello mushrooms.

- In a bowl, mix cooked farro or quinoa, tomatoes, olives, onions, and feta cheese.
- Brush mushrooms with olive oil and season with salt, pepper, and oregano.
- Stuff mushrooms with the farro mixture and place in a baking dish.
- Bake for 20-25 minutes, until mushrooms are tender.
- Serve warm.

5. Spicy Lentil and Kale Stew:

Ingredients:

- 1 cup dried lentils, rinsed
- 1 onion, chopped
- 2 cloves garlic, minced
- 1 large carrot, diced
- 1 celery stalk, diced
- 1 can diced tomatoes

- 4 cups vegetable or chicken broth
- 1 teaspoon ground cumin
- 1/2 teaspoon paprika
- 1/4 teaspoon cayenne pepper (adjust to taste)
- 2 cups chopped kale or spinach
- Salt and pepper to taste

Instructions:

- In a large pot, sauté onion, garlic, carrot, and celery until softened.
- Add lentils, diced tomatoes, broth, cumin, paprika, cayenne pepper, salt, and pepper.
- Bring to a boil, then reduce heat and simmer for 25-30 minutes, until lentils are tender.
- Stir in kale or spinach and cook for another 5 minutes.
- Serve hot.

These dinner recipes are designed to provide iron-rich meals while incorporating vitamin C sources to enhance iron absorption, making them great options for supporting anemia management and overall health.

Snack And Smoothie Recipes

Here are some anemia-friendly snack and smoothie recipes that are rich in iron and vitamin C to support better iron absorption:

Snacks:

1. Greek Yogurt with Berries and Nuts:

Ingredients:

- 1 cup Greek yogurt
- 1/2 cup mixed berries (strawberries, blueberries, raspberries)

- 2 tablespoons chopped nuts (almonds, walnuts)
- 1 teaspoon honey (optional)

Instructions:

- Spoon Greek yogurt into a bowl.
- Top with mixed berries and chopped nuts.
- Drizzle with honey if desired.
- Enjoy as a nutritious snack.

2. Hummus with Veggie Sticks:

Ingredients:

- 1 cup hummus (store-bought or homemade)
- Assorted veggie sticks (carrots, bell peppers, cucumber, celery)

Instructions:

- Arrange veggie sticks on a plate.

- Serve with a side of hummus for dipping.
- Enjoy the crunchy, nutrient-packed snack.

3. Apple Slices with Almond Butter:

Ingredients:

- 1 apple, sliced
- 2 tablespoons almond butter

Instructions:

- Slice the apple into wedges.
- Dip apple slices into almond butter.
- Enjoy this easy and iron-rich snack.

4. Iron-Rich Energy Balls:

Ingredients:

- 1 cup oats
- 1/2 cup nut butter (peanut or almond)
- 1/4 cup honey or maple syrup
- 1/4 cup chia seeds
- 1/4 cup raisins or dried apricots (chopped)
- 1 tablespoon cocoa powder (optional)

Instructions:

- Mix all ingredients in a bowl until well combined.
- Roll mixture into small balls (about 1 inch in diameter).
- Store in an airtight container in the refrigerator for up to a week.

5. Roasted Pumpkin Seeds:

Ingredients:

- 1 cup pumpkin seeds
- 1 tablespoon olive oil
- 1/2 teaspoon smoked paprika
- Salt to taste

Instructions:

- Preheat oven to 350°F (175°C).
- Toss pumpkin seeds with olive oil, smoked paprika, and salt.
- Spread seeds on a baking sheet in a single layer.
- Roast for 10-15 minutes, stirring occasionally, until crispy.
- Allow to cool before eating.

Smoothies:

1. Berry Spinach Smoothie:

Ingredients:

- 1 cup fresh spinach
- 1/2 cup frozen mixed berries (strawberries, blueberries, raspberries)
- 1 banana
- 1 cup fortified plant-based milk or regular milk
- 1 tablespoon chia seeds

Instructions:

- Combine all ingredients in a blender.
- Blend until smooth.
- Pour into a glass and enjoy!

2. Tropical Iron Boost Smoothie:

Ingredients:

- 1/2 cup pineapple chunks (rich in vitamin C)
- 1/2 cup mango chunks
- 1 cup kale
- 1/2 cup Greek yogurt
- 1 tablespoon flaxseeds

Instructions:

- Add all ingredients to a blender.
- Blend until creamy and smooth.
- Serve chilled.

3. Orange and Carrot Smoothie:

Ingredients:

- 1 large orange, peeled
- 1/2 cup carrot juice
- 1/2 cup Greek yogurt

- 1/2 banana
- 1/2 teaspoon ginger (optional)

Instructions:

- Combine all ingredients in a blender.
- Blend until smooth.
- Enjoy this refreshing and vitamin C-rich smoothie.

4. Green Apple and Spinach Smoothie:

Ingredients:

- 1 green apple, cored and chopped
- 1 cup fresh spinach
- 1/2 cucumber, chopped
- 1/2 cup coconut water or water
- 1 tablespoon hemp seeds

Instructions:

- Place all ingredients in a blender.

- Blend until smooth and creamy.
- Pour into a glass and enjoy!

5. Iron-Packed Smoothie Bowl:

Ingredients:

- 1/2 cup frozen mixed berries
- 1/2 cup spinach
- 1/2 cup fortified plant-based milk or regular milk
- 1 tablespoon pumpkin seeds
- 1/4 cup granola (optional)

Instructions:

- Blend frozen berries, spinach, and milk until smooth.
- Pour into a bowl and top with pumpkin seeds and granola.
- Enjoy with a spoon for a satisfying and nutrient-rich snack.

These snacks and smoothies are designed to provide a good balance of iron and vitamin C, helping to support better iron absorption and overall health.

CHAPTER FOUR

Cooking Tips To Maximize Nutrient Retention

Maximizing nutrient retention while cooking is important for maintaining the nutritional value of your meals. Here are some practical tips to help you preserve essential nutrients in your food:

1. Use Minimal Heat:

• **Avoid Overcooking**: Cook vegetables and meats at moderate temperatures and for shorter times to prevent the loss of vitamins and minerals.

• **Steaming Over Boiling**: Steaming vegetables helps retain more nutrients compared to boiling, which can cause nutrients to leach into the cooking water.

2. Opt for Cooking Methods that Preserve Nutrients:

• **Steaming**: Great for vegetables, as it helps retain vitamins and minerals.

• **Sautéing**: Using a small amount of oil to cook food quickly over medium-high heat helps retain nutrients better than boiling.

• **Roasting**: Helps preserve nutrients, particularly in vegetables, when done at moderate temperatures.

3. Minimize Water Usage:

• **Reduce Boiling**: Avoid excessive boiling of vegetables. Use just enough water to cook them or opt for methods like roasting or steaming.

- **Use Cooking Liquids**: If you do boil, use the water in soups or sauces to retain nutrients that may have leached out.

4. Cook with Skin and Peel:

- **Leave Skins On**: Many fruits and vegetables have nutrients in or just under the skin. For example, leave the skin on potatoes and apples where possible.

5. Avoid High Temperatures:

- **Moderate Heat**: High temperatures can degrade certain vitamins. Cook at medium to low heat when possible, especially for nutrients sensitive to heat like vitamin C.

6. Cut Food After Cooking:

- **Cut Larger Pieces**: Cutting vegetables after cooking rather than before can help retain more nutrients. Smaller pieces have more surface area and can lose nutrients more quickly.

7. Preserve Nutrients with Proper Storage:

• **Store Properly**: Store fresh fruits and vegetables in a cool, dark place or the refrigerator to minimize nutrient loss.

• **Use Fresh Ingredients**: The longer fruits and vegetables are stored, the more nutrients they may lose. Use fresh ingredients whenever possible.

8. Use Cookware Wisely:

• **Avoid High-PH Cookware**: Use non-reactive cookware like stainless steel or glass to avoid nutrient loss from reactions with acidic or alkaline foods.

- **Lid on Pots**: Cooking with the lid on can help retain moisture and reduce cooking time, which can preserve nutrients.

9. Consider Soaking and Sprouting:

- **Soak Beans and Grains**: Soaking beans and grains can reduce cooking time and improve nutrient availability.

- **Sprout Seeds**: Sprouting seeds can increase their vitamin content and make them easier to digest.

10. Add Acidic Ingredients Wisely:

- **Add Lemon or Vinegar**: Adding lemon juice or vinegar to dishes can help with the absorption of certain nutrients, like iron, especially when combined with non-heme iron sources.

11. Avoid Excessive Salt:

• **Limit Salt**: Excessive salt can sometimes inhibit nutrient absorption, particularly minerals like calcium. Use herbs and spices for flavor instead.

By applying these cooking tips, you can better preserve the nutritional value of your meals and ensure you get the most benefit from your food.

Combining Foods For Optimal Nutrient Absorption

Combining foods strategically can significantly enhance nutrient absorption and overall health. Here's how to pair foods to maximize nutrient benefits:

1. Iron and Vitamin C:

• **Why It Works**: Vitamin C enhances the absorption of non-heme iron (the type of iron found in plant-based foods).

Pairings:

• **Spinach Salad with Strawberries**: Add strawberries to a spinach salad to boost iron absorption from the spinach.

• **Lentil Soup with Lemon Juice**: Squeeze lemon juice into your lentil soup for a vitamin C boost.

2. Fat-Soluble Vitamins and Healthy Fats:

• **Why It Works**: Vitamins A, D, E, and K are fat-soluble, meaning they require fat for absorption.

Pairings:

• **Carrot Sticks with Hummus**: Pair carrots (rich in vitamin A) with hummus (containing healthy fats) for better absorption.

• **Avocado with Salad**: Add avocado to a salad to enhance the absorption of vitamins A, D, E, and K from the vegetables.

3. Calcium and Vitamin D:

• **Why It Works**: Vitamin D enhances calcium absorption and bone health.

Pairings:

• **Fortified Orange Juice with Dairy or Fortified Plant-Based Milk**: Drink fortified orange juice (vitamin D) with dairy or fortified plant-based milk (calcium) for optimal bone health.

• **Salmon with a Side of Greens**: Salmon (vitamin D) paired with calcium-rich leafy greens can support bone strength.

4. Protein and Iron:

• **Why It Works**: While not as direct as vitamin C and iron, adequate protein intake can support overall blood health.

Pairings:

• **Quinoa with Black Beans**: Combine quinoa and black beans to benefit from both plant-based proteins and iron.

- **Chicken Stir-Fry with Broccoli**: Pair chicken (heme iron) with broccoli (vitamin C) to enhance iron absorption and overall protein intake.

5. Magnesium and Vitamin D:

- **Why It Works**: Magnesium supports vitamin D metabolism, which is crucial for calcium absorption.

Pairings:

- **Almonds with Fortified Milk**: Eat almonds (magnesium) with fortified milk (vitamin D) for enhanced bone health.

- **Spinach Salad with Fortified Yogurt**: Pair spinach (magnesium) with a serving of fortified yogurt (vitamin D).

6. Zinc and Protein:

• **Why It Works**: Protein helps with the absorption of zinc and supports overall immune function.

Pairings:

• **Beef Stir-Fry with Bell Peppers**: Beef (zinc) with bell peppers (vitamin C) can enhance nutrient absorption and overall health.

• **Nuts and Seeds with a Side of Eggs**: Nuts and seeds (zinc) paired with eggs (protein) can support immune health and nutrient absorption.

7. Fiber and Iron:

• **Why It Works**: While fiber can inhibit iron absorption, combining high-fiber foods with vitamin C-rich foods can balance absorption.

Pairings:

• **Whole-Grain Toast with Kiwi**: Whole-grain toast (fiber) with kiwi (vitamin C) can help improve iron absorption.

• **Oatmeal with Berries**: Combine iron-rich oatmeal with vitamin C-rich berries for a balanced breakfast.

8. Antioxidants and Healthy Fats:

• **Why It Works**: Antioxidants from fruits and vegetables are better absorbed when paired with healthy fats.

Pairings:

• **Tomato and Olive Oil**: Pair tomatoes (antioxidants) with olive oil (healthy fats) to enhance the absorption of lycopene.

• **Spinach Salad with Olive Oil Dressing**: Add olive oil to your spinach salad to help absorb antioxidants like beta-carotene.

Tips for Effective Food Combining:

- **Diverse Plates**: Incorporate a variety of foods to ensure you're getting a broad spectrum of nutrients.
- **Balance Meals**: Combine protein, healthy fats, and carbohydrates with nutrient-dense vegetables and fruits.
- **Consider Timing**: Aim to pair nutrient-enhancing foods

throughout the day, not just in one meal.

By thoughtfully combining foods, you can maximize nutrient absorption and support overall health more effectively.

CHAPTER FIVE
Managing Anemia With Vegetarian And Vegan Diets

Managing anemia on a vegetarian or vegan diet involves focusing on plant-based sources of iron and ensuring you're meeting your overall nutritional needs to support healthy red blood cell production. Here's how to effectively manage anemia with vegetarian and vegan diets:

Iron-Rich Plant-Based Foods:

Legumes:

• **Sources**: Lentils, chickpeas, black beans, kidney beans.

• **Example**: Lentil soup, chickpea salad, black bean tacos.

Leafy Greens:

- **Sources**: Spinach, kale, Swiss chard, collard greens.

- **Example**: Spinach salads, kale smoothies, sautéed greens.

Whole Grains:

- **Sources**: Quinoa, brown rice, oatmeal, barley.

- **Example**: Quinoa salad, brown rice stir-fry, oatmeal with fruit.

Nuts and Seeds:

- **Sources**: Pumpkin seeds, sesame seeds, sunflower seeds, almonds.

- **Example**: Pumpkin seed trail mix, almond butter, chia seed pudding.

Fortified Foods:

- **Sources**: Fortified cereals, plant-based milks (e.g., soy, almond), nutritional yeast.

- **Example**: Fortified cereal with berries, plant-based milk in smoothies.

Dried Fruits:

- **Sources**: Apricots, raisins, figs, dates.

- **Example**: Dried fruit snacks, adding to salads or oatmeal.

Enhancing Iron Absorption:

Combine with Vitamin C:

- **Why**: Vitamin C enhances non-heme iron absorption from plant sources.

Examples:

- **Add Citrus Fruits**: Oranges, strawberries, or kiwi to meals.

- **Pair with Vegetables**: Bell peppers, broccoli, or tomatoes.

Avoid Iron Blockers:

- **Why**: Certain substances can inhibit iron absorption.

Examples:

- **Limit Coffee and Tea**: Consume separately from iron-rich meals.

- **Reduce Calcium Intake During Meals**: High calcium foods can compete with iron absorption.

Sample Meal Ideas:

Breakfast:

- **Iron-Fortified Cereal with Berries and Almond Milk**: Choose a cereal fortified with iron and pair with vitamin C-rich berries and fortified almond milk.

Lunch:

- **Chickpea and Spinach Salad**: Combine chickpeas with fresh spinach, bell peppers, cherry tomatoes, and a lemon-tahini dressing.

Dinner:

- **Quinoa and Black Bean Stuffed Bell Peppers**: Stuff bell peppers with quinoa, black beans, corn, and tomatoes. Serve with a side of steamed broccoli.

Snacks:

- **Pumpkin Seeds and Dried Apricots**: A handful of pumpkin seeds and a few dried apricots make a nutrient-dense snack.

- **Smoothie with Spinach and Citrus**: Blend spinach with a banana, orange, and a tablespoon of chia seeds.

Dessert:

- **Chia Seed Pudding with Berries**: Prepare chia seed pudding with fortified plant-based milk and top with vitamin C-rich berries.

Nutritional Considerations:

Vitamin B12:

- **Why**: Essential for red blood cell formation, often lacking in vegan diets.

- **Sources**: Fortified foods (nutritional yeast, fortified plant-based milks) or supplements.

Folate:

- **Why**: Crucial for red blood cell production.

- **Sources**: Leafy greens, legumes, fortified cereals.

Omega-3 Fatty Acids:

- **Why**: Supports overall health and can be low in vegan diets.

- **Sources**: Flaxseeds, chia seeds, hemp seeds, walnuts.

Protein:

- **Why**: Important for overall health and energy.

- **Sources**: Legumes, tofu, tempeh, edamame, quinoa.

Calcium:

- **Why**: Necessary for bone health and can affect iron absorption.

- **Sources**: Fortified plant-based milks, tofu, leafy greens.

Tips for Success:

- **Regular Monitoring**: Regularly check your iron levels and adjust your diet or supplements as needed.
- **Varied Diet**: Incorporate a wide variety of foods to cover all essential nutrients.
- **Consultation**: Work with a healthcare provider or dietitian to

ensure your dietary needs are met and to get personalized advice.

By focusing on iron-rich plant foods, enhancing absorption with vitamin C, and managing other nutritional needs, you can effectively manage anemia on a vegetarian or vegan diet.

Hydration And Its Role In Anemia Management

Hydration plays a crucial role in overall health and can be an important factor in managing anemia. Here's how staying properly hydrated can impact anemia and some tips on maintaining adequate hydration:

Importance of Hydration in Anemia Management

Maintaining Blood Volume:

- **Why It Matters**: Adequate hydration helps maintain blood volume and circulation. Proper blood volume supports efficient oxygen transport and nutrient delivery to tissues, which is vital for individuals with anemia.

- **Effect**: Dehydration can lead to reduced blood volume, making anemia symptoms more pronounced and potentially impacting overall health.

Supporting Red Blood Cell Production:

- **Why It Matters**: Proper hydration supports the function of the kidneys and bone marrow, which are involved in red blood cell production and regulation.

- **Effect**: Adequate fluid intake helps maintain kidney function, which is crucial for the production of erythropoietin, a hormone that stimulates red blood cell production.

Enhancing Nutrient Absorption:

- **Why It Matters**: Hydration helps with the digestion and absorption of nutrients, including iron, vitamin C, and folate.

- **Effect**: Proper hydration can enhance the absorption of iron and other essential nutrients needed to manage anemia effectively.

Preventing Dehydration-Related Symptoms:

- **Why It Matters**: Dehydration can exacerbate symptoms of anemia, such as fatigue, dizziness, and weakness.

- **Effect**: Staying hydrated helps mitigate these symptoms and supports overall well-being.

Tips for Maintaining Adequate Hydration:

Drink Enough Fluids:

- **Guideline**: Aim for about 8 cups (2 liters) of water per day, though individual needs may vary based on activity level, climate, and health status.

- **Hydration Sources**: Include water, herbal teas, and low-sugar fruit juices.

Include Hydrating Foods:

- **Examples**: Eat foods with high water content, such as cucumbers, celery, watermelon, and oranges, which also provide additional nutrients and hydration.

Monitor Fluid Intake:

- **Tracking**: Keep track of your fluid intake and ensure you're meeting your hydration needs throughout the day.

Adjust for Activity and Climate:

- **Exercise**: Increase fluid intake with physical activity to replace lost fluids.

- **Climate**: Drink more fluids in hot or dry climates to compensate for increased water loss through sweat.

Limit Dehydrating Beverages:

- **Examples**: Minimize intake of caffeinated and alcoholic beverages, as they can increase fluid loss and contribute to dehydration.

Watch for Signs of Dehydration:

- **Symptoms**: Pay attention to signs such as dark urine, dizziness, dry mouth, and fatigue. Address these symptoms promptly by increasing fluid intake.

Balance Electrolytes:

- **Importance**: Ensure you're getting enough electrolytes (sodium, potassium) through a balanced diet, especially if you're consuming large amounts of water, to avoid electrolyte imbalances.

Incorporating Hydration into Meals

Start with a Hydrating Breakfast:

- **Example**: Include a smoothie made with fruits and leafy greens or a bowl of oatmeal topped with fresh fruit and nuts.

Hydrating Soups and Stews:

• **Example**: Enjoy brothy soups or stews that provide both hydration and nutrients.

Healthy Snacks:

• **Example**: Snack on hydrating fruits like apples or berries and include a glass of water or herbal tea.

By maintaining proper hydration, you support various bodily functions that can aid in managing anemia, enhance nutrient absorption, and overall health.

CHAPTER SIX'
When To Consider Supplements & Choosing The Right Supplements

When managing anemia, supplements can be beneficial, particularly when dietary intake alone may not be sufficient to meet your nutritional needs. Here's a guide on when to consider supplements and how to choose the right ones:

When to Consider Supplements

Diagnosis of Deficiency:

• **Reason**: If you have been diagnosed with an iron deficiency or other specific nutrient deficiencies, supplements may be necessary to correct the imbalance.

• **Action**: Consult with a healthcare provider for a proper diagnosis and treatment plan.

Dietary Limitations:

• **Reason**: If your diet lacks variety or certain key nutrients (e.g., iron, vitamin B12) due to dietary restrictions (e.g., vegetarian or vegan diet), supplements can help fill nutritional gaps.

• **Action**: Evaluate your diet and consult with a dietitian or healthcare provider to determine if supplements are needed.

Chronic Health Conditions:

• **Reason**: Conditions that affect nutrient absorption (e.g., celiac disease, Crohn's disease) may necessitate supplements to meet nutritional needs.

• **Action**: Work with a healthcare provider to manage your condition and address nutrient deficiencies.

Symptoms of Deficiency:

- **Reason**: Symptoms such as fatigue, weakness, pallor, or dizziness may indicate a nutrient deficiency that could benefit from supplementation.

- **Action**: Consult with a healthcare provider for a proper evaluation and supplement recommendations.

Pregnancy or Lactation:

- **Reason**: Pregnant or breastfeeding women have increased nutritional needs, and supplements may be necessary to support both maternal and infant health.

- **Action**: Follow healthcare provider recommendations for prenatal or postnatal supplements.

Choosing the Right Supplements:

Iron Supplements:

- **Forms**: Ferrous sulfate, ferrous gluconate, ferrous fumarate.

- **Considerations**: Choose a form of iron that is well-absorbed and easy on the stomach. Iron supplements can sometimes cause gastrointestinal issues, so starting with a lower dose and gradually increasing can help.

- **Vitamin C**: Taking iron supplements with vitamin C can enhance absorption. Some iron supplements come combined with vitamin C.

Vitamin B12 Supplements:

- **Forms**: Cyanocobalamin, methylcobalamin.

- **Considerations**: Vegans and those with absorption issues may need B12 supplements. Methylcobalamin is often preferred for its better absorption.

Folate Supplements:

- **Forms**: Folic acid (synthetic), methylfolate (bioactive form).

- **Considerations**: Folate is crucial for red blood cell production. Methylfolate is the active form and may be better absorbed by some individuals.

Vitamin D Supplements:

- **Forms**: Vitamin D2 (ergocalciferol), Vitamin D3 (cholecalciferol).

- **Considerations**: Vitamin D3 is generally more effective at raising blood levels of vitamin D. Essential for calcium absorption and bone health.

Multivitamins:

• **Considerations**: If you have multiple deficiencies or need general support, a well-rounded multivitamin can help provide essential nutrients. Look for one with balanced iron levels and minimal fillers.

Omega-3 Fatty Acids:

• **Forms**: Fish oil, algae oil.

• **Considerations**: Omega-3s support overall health. For vegans, algae oil is a plant-based option.

Calcium Supplements:

- **Forms**: Calcium carbonate, calcium citrate.

- **Considerations**: Calcium citrate is better absorbed, especially in individuals with lower stomach acid. Avoid taking calcium supplements at the same time as iron supplements, as calcium can inhibit iron absorption.

Tips for Choosing Supplements

Consult a Healthcare Provider:

- **Reason**: A healthcare provider can assess your specific needs, recommend appropriate supplements, and ensure there are no interactions with other medications or conditions.

- **Action**: Discuss your health status and dietary intake with a healthcare provider before starting any new supplements.

Check for Quality:

- **Reason**: Quality can vary between brands. Choose supplements that are third-party tested for purity and potency.

- **Action**: Look for certifications or seals of approval from reputable organizations.

Avoid Over-Supplementation:

- **Reason**: Excessive intake of certain nutrients can be harmful. Follow recommended dosages and avoid taking multiple supplements with overlapping nutrients.

- **Action**: Monitor total nutrient intake from all sources to prevent exceeding safe levels.

Consider Bioavailability:

- **Reason**: The form of the supplement can impact how well it is absorbed and utilized by the body.

- **Action**: Opt for supplements in forms that are known for better bioavailability.

By understanding when to consider supplements and selecting the right ones, you can more effectively manage anemia and support your overall health.

Tracking Symptoms And Progress

Tracking symptoms and progress is essential for managing anemia effectively. It helps you and your healthcare provider assess how well your treatment plan is working and make necessary adjustments. Here's a guide on how to track your symptoms and progress:

1. Keep a Symptom Diary:

Why It's Important:

- **Identifies Patterns**: Helps recognize patterns or triggers that affect your symptoms.

- **Provides Insight**: Gives a clearer picture of how your anemia is impacting your daily life.

How to Do It:

- **Daily Log**: Record symptoms daily, noting their severity and any associated factors (e.g., time of day, recent meals).

- **Details**: Include details like fatigue levels, dizziness, weakness, paleness, and any other relevant symptoms.

- **Triggers**: Note any potential triggers such as changes in diet, stress levels, or physical activity.

2. Monitor Dietary Intake:

Why It's Important:

- **Nutrient Intake**: Ensures you're consuming enough iron, vitamin C, and other essential nutrients.

- **Identifies Deficiencies**: Helps identify if dietary changes are needed.

How to Do It:

• **Food Diary**: Record everything you eat and drink, including portion sizes.

• **Track Nutrients**: Use apps or journals to track iron-rich foods and other relevant nutrients.

• **Review and Adjust**: Regularly review your intake to ensure you're meeting your nutritional needs.

3. Track Supplement Usage

Why It's Important:

• **Consistency**: Ensures you're taking your supplements as prescribed.

• **Effectiveness**: Helps evaluate the effectiveness of supplements in managing your anemia.

How to Do It:

- **Schedule**: Create a schedule for taking supplements and stick to it.

- **Record**: Note the type, dosage, and frequency of each supplement.

- **Monitor Effects**: Record any side effects or changes in symptoms related to supplement intake.

4. Monitor Vital Signs:

Why It's Important:

- **Health Status**: Provides insights into how anemia is affecting your overall health.

- **Early Detection**: Helps detect any worsening of symptoms or new health issues.

How to Do It:

• **Regular Check-Ups**: Have regular check-ups with your healthcare provider to monitor vital signs such as blood pressure and heart rate.

• **Home Monitoring**: If advised, use home monitoring devices to track vital signs and symptoms.

5. Track Blood Work Results

Why It's Important:

• **Assess Progress**: Helps evaluate how well your treatment is working and if your anemia is improving.

• **Adjust Treatment**: Allows for adjustments to your treatment plan based on lab results.

How to Do It:

- **Record Results**: Keep a record of your blood test results, including hemoglobin levels, ferritin, and other relevant markers.

- **Review Trends**: Look for trends in your results over time to assess progress.

6. Set Goals and Review Progress

Why It's Important:

- **Motivation**: Helps stay motivated by setting achievable goals.

- **Adjustment**: Allows you to make informed decisions about changes to your treatment plan.

How to Do It:

- **Set Short-Term Goals**: Set achievable short-term goals such as increasing iron intake or reducing symptoms.

- **Review Regularly**: Regularly review your progress towards these goals and adjust as needed.

7. Communicate with Your Healthcare Provider:

Why It's Important:

- **Collaboration**: Ensures that your treatment plan is on track and allows for timely adjustments.

Feedback: Provides valuable feedback for improving your management plan.

How to Do It:

- **Regular Updates**: Share your symptom diary, dietary logs, and any changes in your health with your healthcare provider.

Discuss Changes: Talk about any significant changes or concerns regarding your anemia management.

By effectively tracking symptoms, dietary intake, supplement usage, and blood work, you can better manage anemia and work with your healthcare provider to optimize your treatment plan.

Regular Blood Tests And What They Mean

Regular blood tests are crucial for monitoring anemia and assessing overall health. They provide detailed information about your blood's composition and how well your body is responding to treatment. Here's an overview of common blood tests related to anemia and what the results mean:

1. Complete Blood Count (CBC)

- **Purpose**: Provides an overview of your overall health and can help diagnose anemia and other conditions.

Key Components:

- **Hemoglobin (Hb or Hgb)**: Measures the amount of hemoglobin in the blood. Low levels can indicate anemia.

- **Hematocrit (Hct)**: Indicates the percentage of blood volume occupied by red blood cells. Low levels suggest anemia.

- **Red Blood Cell Count (RBC)**: Measures the number of red blood cells in a given volume of blood. Low RBC can be a sign of anemia.

- **Mean Corpuscular Volume (MCV)**: Measures the average size of red blood cells. Low MCV (microcytic) can indicate iron deficiency anemia, while high MCV (macrocytic) can suggest vitamin B12 or folate deficiency.

- **Mean Corpuscular Hemoglobin (MCH)**: Indicates the average amount of hemoglobin per red blood cell. Low MCH may be associated with iron deficiency.

- **Mean Corpuscular Hemoglobin Concentration (MCHC)**: Measures the concentration of hemoglobin in red blood cells. Low MCHC can be indicative of anemia.

2. Serum Iron

- **Purpose**: Measures the amount of iron in the blood. It helps assess iron levels and diagnose iron deficiency anemia.

Interpretation:

- **Low Levels**: May indicate iron deficiency anemia or chronic disease.

- **Normal or High Levels**: May suggest other types of anemia or conditions affecting iron metabolism.

3. Ferritin

• **Purpose**: Measures the amount of stored iron in the body. Ferritin levels can indicate how much iron is available for producing red blood cells.

Interpretation:

• **Low Ferritin**: Often indicates iron deficiency anemia.

• **Normal or High Ferritin**: May suggest anemia of chronic disease or other conditions affecting iron storage.

4. Total Iron-Binding Capacity (TIBC)

• **Purpose**: Measures the blood's capacity to bind and transport iron. It helps in diagnosing iron deficiency anemia.

Interpretation:

• **High TIBC**: Often seen in iron deficiency anemia, indicating that the body is trying to increase iron transport.

• **Low TIBC**: Can be associated with anemia of chronic disease or other conditions affecting iron metabolism.

5. Transferrin Saturation

• **Purpose**: Measures the percentage of transferrin (a protein that binds iron) that is saturated with iron. It helps evaluate iron availability and absorption.

Interpretation:

• **Low Saturation**: Often indicates iron deficiency anemia.

- **Normal or High Saturation**: Can suggest other types of anemia or iron overload conditions.

6. Vitamin B12 and Folate Levels

- **Purpose**: Measures levels of vitamin B12 and folate, which are essential for red blood cell production and DNA synthesis.

Interpretation:

- **Low Vitamin B12**: Can indicate vitamin B12 deficiency anemia or absorption issues.

- **Low Folate**: Often associated with folate deficiency anemia, which can be caused by poor diet or absorption issues.

7. Reticulocyte Count

- **Purpose**: Measures the number of young red blood cells (reticulocytes) in the blood. It helps assess bone marrow function and the body's response to anemia.

Interpretation:

- **High Reticulocyte Count**: Indicates that the bone marrow is producing more red blood cells in response to anemia.

- **Low Reticulocyte Count**: Suggests that the bone marrow is not producing enough red blood cells, which can be due to various types of anemia or bone marrow disorders.

8. Erythrocyte Sedimentation Rate (ESR) or C-Reactive Protein (CRP)

• **Purpose**: Measures inflammation levels in the body. Inflammatory conditions can affect anemia.

Interpretation:

- **Elevated ESR or CRP**: Indicates inflammation or chronic disease, which can affect anemia and its management.

9. Liver Function Tests

• **Purpose**: Assesses liver health, which can impact iron metabolism and anemia management.

Interpretation:

• **Abnormal Levels**: May indicate liver disease or conditions affecting iron metabolism and storage.

10. Kidney Function Tests

• **Purpose**: Evaluates kidney function, which is important for red blood cell production and overall health.

Interpretation:

• **Abnormal Levels**: Can affect erythropoietin production, a hormone that stimulates red blood cell production.

Regular Monitoring:

• **Frequency**: The frequency of blood tests depends on your specific condition and treatment plan. It may be weekly, monthly, or as directed by your healthcare provider.

• **Communication**: Share test results with your healthcare provider to assess progress, adjust treatment plans, and address any concerns.

By understanding and monitoring these blood tests, you can better manage anemia, track treatment effectiveness, and make informed decisions about your health.

CHAPTER SEVEN
Adjusting Your Diet Based On Test Results

Adjusting your diet based on blood test results is essential for effectively managing anemia and improving overall health. Here's a guide on how to tailor your diet according to various test results:

1. Low Hemoglobin or Hematocrit

- **Indicates**: Possible anemia or low red blood cell count.

Dietary Adjustments:

- **Increase Iron-Rich Foods**: Focus on foods high in heme iron (from animal sources) or non-heme iron (from plant sources). Examples include red meat, poultry, fish, lentils, beans, and fortified cereals.

- **Enhance Iron Absorption**: Include vitamin C-rich foods (e.g., citrus fruits, bell peppers) with iron-rich meals to improve absorption.

2. Low Serum Iron

- **Indicates**: Iron deficiency anemia or inadequate iron stores.

Dietary Adjustments:

- **Boost Iron Intake**: Increase consumption of iron-rich foods like spinach, tofu, and quinoa.

- **Consider Iron Supplements**: If dietary changes are insufficient, supplements may be necessary, as advised by your healthcare provider.

3. Low Ferritin

- **Indicates**: Depleted iron stores, often seen in iron deficiency anemia.

Dietary Adjustments:

- **Increase Iron-Rich Foods**: Prioritize iron-rich foods and consider cooking in cast-iron pans to boost iron intake.

- **Combine with Vitamin C**: Eat vitamin C-rich foods alongside iron-rich meals to enhance iron absorption.

4. High Total Iron-Binding Capacity (TIBC)

- **Indicates**: Often associated with iron deficiency anemia.

Dietary Adjustments:

• **Focus on Iron Intake**: Increase intake of iron-rich foods and ensure adequate absorption by pairing with vitamin C-rich foods.

• **Avoid Calcium and Caffeine Around Meals**: Minimize intake of calcium and caffeinated beverages during iron-rich meals as they can inhibit iron absorption.

5. Low Transferrin Saturation

• **Indicates**: Low iron availability or possible iron deficiency.

Dietary Adjustments:

• **Enhance Iron Absorption**: Focus on iron-rich foods and combine them with vitamin C sources to improve absorption.

- **Avoid Iron Blockers**: Limit substances like calcium, coffee, and tea around iron-rich meals.

6. Low Vitamin B12

- **Indicates**: Vitamin B12 deficiency, which can lead to anemia.

Dietary Adjustments:

- **Increase B12 Sources**: Include more vitamin B12-rich foods like eggs, dairy products, and fortified plant-based milks. Vegans may need fortified foods or supplements.

- **Consult Your Provider**: Consider vitamin B12 supplements if dietary sources are insufficient or absorption is an issue.

7. Low Folate

• **Indicates**: Folate deficiency, which can cause anemia.

Dietary Adjustments:

• **Increase Folate-Rich Foods**: Incorporate foods high in folate, such as leafy greens, legumes, and fortified cereals.

• **Consider Folate Supplements**: If dietary intake is inadequate or if there are absorption issues, supplements may be necessary.

8. High Erythrocyte Sedimentation Rate (ESR) or C-Reactive Protein (CRP)

• **Indicates**: Inflammation or chronic disease affecting anemia.

Dietary Adjustments:

- **Anti-Inflammatory Foods**: Focus on foods with anti-inflammatory properties, such as fatty fish, nuts, seeds, fruits, and vegetables.

- **Manage Chronic Conditions**: Address any underlying conditions that may be contributing to inflammation and anemia.

9. Abnormal Liver Function Tests

- **Indicates**: Possible liver issues affecting iron metabolism.

Dietary Adjustments:

- **Support Liver Health**: Include liver-friendly foods such as leafy greens, beets, and foods rich in antioxidants.

- **Limit Alcohol**: Avoid or limit alcohol intake as it can affect liver function and overall health.

10. Abnormal Kidney Function Tests

- **Indicates**: Potential kidney issues that could impact red blood cell production.

Dietary Adjustments:

- **Support Kidney Health**: Focus on a balanced diet low in sodium and protein to reduce strain on the kidneys.

- **Consult a Dietitian**: Work with a dietitian to tailor your diet based on kidney function and overall health needs.

General Tips for Adjusting Your Diet:

- **Consult Healthcare Professionals**: Always work with a healthcare provider or dietitian to make informed dietary changes based on your blood test results.

- **Monitor Changes**: Track how dietary adjustments impact your symptoms and blood test results over time.

- **Stay Informed**: Keep updated on nutritional needs and make adjustments as needed based on ongoing test results and health status.

By aligning your diet with your test results, you can better manage anemia, support your overall health, and optimize the effectiveness of your treatment plan.

Managing anemia effectively involves a comprehensive approach that includes understanding the condition, adjusting dietary habits, and closely monitoring progress through regular blood tests.

It is possible to effectively manage anemia, improve your overall well-being, and improve your quality of life by implementing a comprehensive approach that encompasses professional guidance, regular monitoring, and proper dietary management.

THE END

www.ingramcontent.com/pod-product-compliance
Lightning Source LLC
Chambersburg PA
CBHW052303220526
45471CB00001B/473